Hanjo Koch

WORKING ON A NEW ME

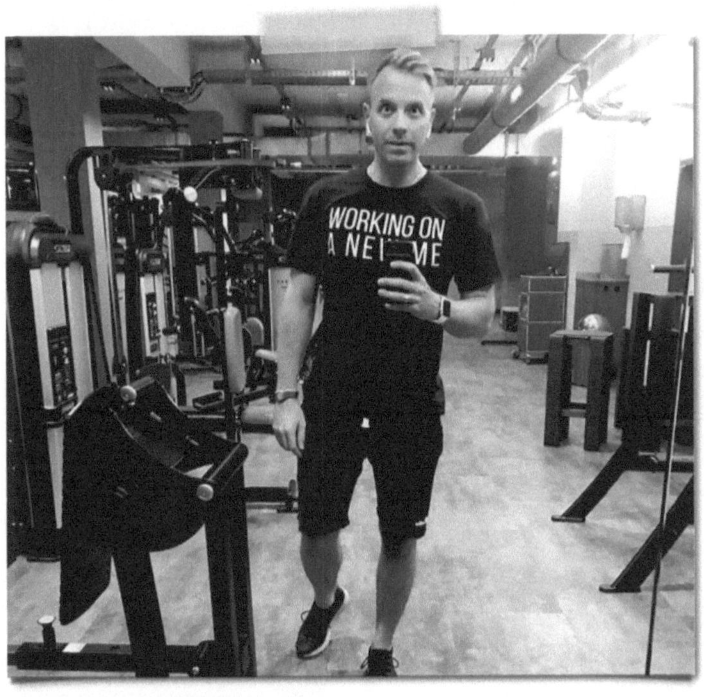

How I reached my fitness goal –
and how a healthy lifestyle
affected my job as well

How I reached my fitness goal – and how a healthy lifestyle affected my job as well.

1st edition | First published in 2020 in ebook form in English language exclusively on Amazon Kindle.

Reading time: 2.5-3.0 hours

Can you relate to this?

Imagine this: You're at a turning point in your life where you realise that some kind of change should happen. And it should happen sooner than later. Because you're already months into the year, and your New Year's resolutions have long been neglected. Or you've started several times, again and again – and truthfully gave up upon it completely. "What's the point anyway?"

Let me show you which path I took from here on, why I came to setting myself a fitness goal, how I reached that goal after quite some time, why giving up was not a feasible option – and how turning to a healthy lifestyle affected my professional life as well, and more than I initially had even thought of.

What began as self-written blog entries turned into full chapters over the months, as I wanted to take you on my journey and share my story with you. You can use the same approaches and ideas I did to make a similar transformation in your life. So why not go ahead and write your own story? I am still on it, by the way, with no intention of quitting or changing my attitude and lifestyle.

This book is not explaining scientifi cally proven studies in detail, there is plenty of literature available in stores and libraries for that. It is intended solely as a motivational read for fi tness and nutrition novices seeking inspiration, wanting to look at 'the guy from next door' and how he did it.

'Working on a new me' reflects my own personal experiences, so remember this can vary for you depending on your own current circumstances, physique, mindset, lifestyle, and the company you keep – so please don't see this book as an ultimate blueprint.

Bonus material: the last weeks of my progress were heavily influenced by a worldwide 'game changer' called COVID-19. I will show you how I coped both privately and professionally with the lockdown and social restrictions due to the corona virus outbreak. And how I did not want to give up achieving my goal.

CHAPTERS:

1. CHOICES: Buying new suits vs. getting in shape again

So I was at that point in life where I repeatedly started feeling uncomfortable in my suits – due to me getting way larger than the size I should wear – and I really needed to take a closer look. Being a sales person, I came to asking myself a possibly familiar question: how many suits do I actually own in my closet?

‚Why suits?' you might ask now. Well, in my profession they are my business attire, I wear them every office day. And I'm required to buy them myself as they are not an official uniform for us.

To be honest, my wardrobe has 5 differently coloured business suits in it, to get me through the weeks without making myself or my co-workers feel bored by my attire. Roughly taking 150 € per suit into account, these outfits alone calculate to approximately 750 € of total value.

‚Do I really want to spend 750 € in one batch?' I asked myself. A whopping 750 Euros for completely new business outfits, leading me to consecutive questions like:

- What shall I do with 5 grown out suits? Sell them second hand? Keep them for when I'm back in my previous shape? They are worth quite a sum if you look at it this way.

- What if I keep getting slightly larger and uncomfortable over time again? Shall I then just buy another batch of suits? For another 750 €? How long will this go on afterwards, and do I actually have the budget for this wardrobe renewal every time?

- What else can I do instead with a "new" budget of 750 € at hand? How about buying a top brand smartphone, making that well deserved week's vacation, fly to visit the family spontaneously – OR make an investment into myself by getting back in my previous shape again?

Well, you don't have to guess what my decision at this point was. But what helped me choose this path? It was weighing different alternatives, each with smaller costs, against the initial 750 Euros, and then comparing them in a timeline until the budget is used up.

Here are some of my examples for how long 750 € could last:

- Gym (fitness centre) @ low budget membership: 15 € per month –> 50 months / 4 years

- Gym @ premium membership: 50 € per month –> 15 months / 1 year + 1 quarter

- Swimming in communal pool: 5 € per visit –> 150 visits / 1 visit per week –> 37 months / 3 years

- Buying healthy (but often more expensive) groceries and fruits: 5 € per shopping / 3 times shopping per week –> 50 weeks / almost 1 year

- Tennis: 13 € for a half court, once per month –> 57 months / 4 years + 9 months

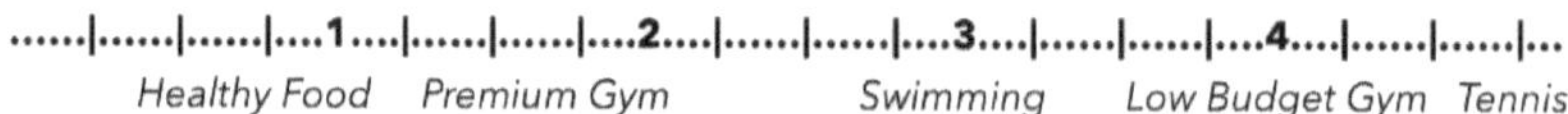

Between one and almost 5 years? Wow, that was a game changer! That gave me many choices! And I didn't take long to get started, get up from that comfortable sofa, and sign a new contract with myself and my goal. **I had decided to #justdoit.**

5 Learnings from this chapter:

1. Make yourself clear what alternatives you could have.

2. Monetise each alternative roughly compared to the initial costs of option one.

3. Write them all down if necessary to compare and weigh against.

4. Transpose them into a timeline to visualise how short or long each would last.

5. Decide and then set up a contract with yourself, fixing the initial costs as your new contractual budget.

2. JUST DO IT: Sign a goal contract with yourself

With my first goal set: ‚Getting in shape again' I now had to be more concise on how I wanted to reach this goal. So I set up a contract with myself. My contract was valid for one year, with a value of the before mentioned 750 €. The small print included a no opt-out paragraph as well as an automatic renewal clause if I were successful.

This way I made sure I would stick to it, not quit by giving up early, and plan ahead by keeping the habit if I enjoyed the results. **Why did it have to be a contract**, you might ask? Think of a basketball player signing up for, say, the Lakers. Or a soccer player transferring into a new season with, say, FC Bayern. On normal grounds they want to finish the season with the best possible team result, working hard to achieve this goal, not thinking about a transfer before the season's end at all.

I was also looking for long-term results, that would require dedication over a time span, that would have me get off the couch and get moving in order to reach my goal. I did not expect it to be easy, and with normal spare time while working a full job I was calculating with **one year until I could see great results**. From previous experience I knew that first results usually show quickly, but that the body wouldn't change in the same speed further on. The desired transformation would therefore need that budget of 750 € assigned and sealed, and I restricted myself from touching it - no matter what!

What could I have used a couple hundred Euros for easily instead?

- A new smartphone,

- Shopping new clothes,

- Dining out more or simply consuming more.

But the contract with myself had the **focus on investing the money in myself**. It made me the centre of my attention, I was my own first priority. It was the commitment I made on what I want to achieve, how I want to achieve it and what my budget would be. I created a powerful motivator which had a big weight of importance too. **I was very clear about my personal goals**, and it helped me big time in sticking to it and keep working on that new me.

Although I myself didn't actually write the contract down, if you prefer to do so this is what it could look like:

Self Contract 'Getting in shape again'

I ________________ hereby commit to follow the below guidelines to the very best of my abilities. I agree to work towards getting in shape again and living a healthier lifestyle. I understand that to achieve this goal I choose to be in charge of my own behaviour and decisions, and I will do what's most important to me. I will take massive action towards my own success and will not lay the blame on others if things don't go as expected. In doing so I shall comply with the terms of this contract.

This contract starts on________________________ and continues until ____________________.
It will automatically renew itself for the same length of time unless the goal is reached prior to the agreed end date.

Current stage on start date: ____

State of change on finish date (goal): ____

Steps and resources needed: ____

Budget assigned to reach goal: _______________ €

In case some or all parts are not met, I agree with the following penalties:

Every time I _______________, I will post my failure online in a social media post or story.
Every time I _______________, I will publicly promise to _______________ within two days.

Mini goal no. 1: _______________________________ I will reward myself with: _______________
Mini goal no. 2: _______________________________ I will reward myself with: _______________
Mini goal no. 3: _______________________________ I will reward myself with: _______________

Signed: _______________ Name: ______________________________ Date: _______________

Witness: _______________ Name: ______________________________ Date: _______________

Did you see the penalties I included in the contract? And why, you might ask? Well, if something hurts I'm very likely not to do it again - or at least not too often. If I set up my own penalty rule, I can choose how painful it really will be for me. Here's an example:

- If I set the rule of posting a photo of my rule breaking, then I can choose to only post an Instagram story that will delete itself anyway after 24 hours. Won't hurt that long.

- When the rules were made by someone else, like a friend, they could hurt much more. If the friend defines that I have to post a permanent posting, my feelings might get hurt more because it might make me more vulnerable.

- On the other hand you could define yourself that permanent posts are the rule, and you could use them as confident progression step-stones, showing truly yourself, without filters, not leaving any downsides out.

Rewards shouldn't be left out either, by the way! If you break down the progress into a few steps and the mini goals you want to achieve along the way, it will help you in visualising your goals better. Take a hike up a mountain, for example:

- If you research the trail in advance and make out 3 resting points (e.g. a bench with a great view, a small café or snack bar to recharge, and a restaurant hut with hot food and drinks near the top) the hike won't appear so exhausting anymore, am I right?

5 Learnings from this chapter:

1. Write down your goal and make a commitment with yourself.

2. Set up a self contract for it in order to stay focused.

3. Plan a budget you won't touch for other things.

4. Plan on rewarding yourself along the journey.

5. Make yourself the priority of your investment.

Optional: If you like, show me copies of your own filled-out contracts by posting them in an Instagram story and tagging me (@hanjokoch).

3. SUMMER BODIES ARE MADE IN WINTER: Or are they not?

A popular belief is that summer bodies are made in winter only. Or that January is the best month to start that gym subscription if you want to succeed before that planned beach vacation. Or that running outside needs warm spring or summer temperatures, which in return would make it impossible to start doing sports in winter, wouldn't it? Which would leave too few time to reach your goal if you started around May or June. And starting after the summer vacation would be no point because it were too late … Or that starting a New Years resolution in the months between February and December won't have any good effect, and you're likely to fail at it anyway.

If it sounds familiar to you, let me take you onto my own journey - which I started toward the end of the year: in December 2017.

For a start, running outside in winter seemed impossible to me: it was wet and cold at that time of year, and hey there'd be snow ahead at some point as well. It simply looked impossible to do with the clothes I had in my wardrobe, I just didn't have the right gear - **or did I?** My old mindset would have ticked it off as impossible, period. My new mindset however got me asking Google for help: 'What clothes should I wear for jogging …

- … in winter

- … in cold weather

- … in the rain

- … in the cold' were its choice of popular search engine questions to choose from.

There seemed to be more people on this planet who seek solutions to similar issues like mine. There were answers out there that showed me that nothing is completely impossible. Or with the words of Albert Einstein: **"Everyone knew it was impossible, until a fool who didn't know came along - and did it."**

I purposely didn't wait a couple of weeks until it was the new year finally. Instead I wanted to get my ass of the sofa **before** all that turkey and Christmas roast could settle around my waist. Why wait if I could just do it? Who needed to give me the approval other then myself? **"Because it matters <u>for who</u> you're doing it** - and that would be yourself" were my new inner thoughts. No one told me to get in shape again - I wanted it! I was the one who signed the contract with myself. I had to start and get going.

Here I was, at the end of the year, with weeks gone of having eaten advent cookies at home and in the office regularly. With evenings of mulled wine and matching fast food consumed on various Christmas markets with colleagues and friends. With holidays of even more cookies plus 3 full Christmas meals per day still ahead of me. With plenty of alcohol to celebrate into the New Year. And with obviously too many reasons to even think of starting at all, am I right?

But here came the surprise: By not procrastinating the start I was about to **finish that year with more fitness levels reached** than I had throughout all the 11 months prior! Simply because I got my bum up, something I didn't manage all year. Because I got up straight away, I didn't postpone the starting point this time around. I wanted to prove myself that results showed as soon as I started, that any sport is better than no sports at all. **That doing is like wanting to - just more badass**.

Truth said, for me it turned out to being a pretty easy way to be better than before - 'cos its NOT about being THE BEST, **it's about being BETTER THAN you were YESTERDAY!**

And once I had started I already asked myself why the hell I hadn't started it all earlier? Why not start in autumn/fall already? Why not in summer when it was warm outside? Why did I find so many excuses before, anyway? Why ...?

5 Learnings from this chapter:

1. Don't wait for the perfect moment: the time is NOW.

2. Start your journey whenever you want, don't wait for or rely on others.

3. If you think it's impossible, google if someone else somewhere maybe already dit it.

4. Stop planning and wanting to - start doing things.

5. You already achieved something great if today you were better than yesterday.

4. RUN, FOREST, RUN: Cardio vs. weights

In the beginning of my journey I was convinced that I found the best option for my getting healthier: **jogging** could be done **anytime** (after work, on a Sunday morning, even as an alternative way to commuting home) and **anywhere** (where I live, during business trips, even a run along the beach sidewalk on vacation). And it was the option involving a relatively small to medium budget for equipment needed (no need for monthly binding contracts, existing shoes and clothes already in the wardrobe, only a few updates on functional underwear and sportswear needed in my case).

I loved jogging for many more reasons: I didn't have to concentrate that much while running - compared to a treadmill where one step too far left could get me falling off and hurting me badly. 😌 After a while my mind could "switch off" and I'd get rid of stress, tension or something big that was on my mind and bugging me. I loved running while listening to music, and finding songs with same/similar beat like my pace, for that started a kind of momentum that could get me run a bit faster or even longer when "I am really in it".

And I could always see a physical challenge achieved, simply with the distance I did: five kilometres, for example, weren't bad to finish (equals 3.1 miles) - and **5 km were a kind of "fitness currency"** many people were familiar with: The 5k road races are the shortest of the most common road running competitions; next are 10 k, half-marathon (21.1 k) and marathon 42.2 k). Compare them with, say, US dollar notes and you'll agree that with 5 $ you can already buy some stuff (10, 20 and 50 $ surely will get you more) and that you're quite familiar with what you can buy for it. Same for me was with the 5 k distance - very relatable when achieved. Practically, **5 k is almost exactly the length of New York's Central Park** - up Fifth Avenue from the pond past the zoo, past the lake and the Guggenheim Museum, and up to the Harlem Meer - if you need a famous measurement relation.

I came to a point though where I was proud of the overall fitness level I had enhanced, but realised I would come towards a turning point soon: a junction with two road signs:

- Cardio / No more progress (straight ahead)

- What's the use anyway (next exit right).

The one keeping me on my current track, but only passing by my real goal as if it were a tourist attraction in the distance. The other one tempting me to give up and agreeing with beliefs like "don't know why I thought it would help" and "told you it won't work for you anyway".

Who said I only had these two choices ahead of me in my journey? Imagine this picture: a single step in a new direction can start a new path and create a pathway if used repeatedly. Bending some grass roots and starting my own new path towards progress - I was ready for it and open for new options.

Along my ‚working-on-a-new-me' timeline, I was only 5 months into the lifestyle change process of incorporating regular cardio workouts. But I realised that it was time to up my motivation level, see faster results and a brighter light at the end of the tunnel.

In fact, **I was open to advice on the ideal fitness programs for me**. Advice I took from the professionals in a gym, who based their input on the needs and goals I expressed. My program can be summarised like this:

• Weight lifting will increase muscle mass which will increase the body's fat burning.

• Weights won't necessarily turn me into having a bodybuilder or Hulk physique, but can get me looking more defined and with an overall healthier appearance.

• The gym can assist me more effectively in seeing more results in my progress.

All of that had me starting a new chapter: I went for a consultation, got a guest pass for a trial period, and signed up to a gym membership in May 2018.

5 Learnings from this chapter:

1. Jogging is a rather inexpensive start to get you going.

2. You can run almost anywhere you are - so no excuses. 😉

3. Weight lifting will bring faster results in fat burning, though.

4. Not everyone will automatically look like a Hulk or a Schwarzenegger.

5. The gym was catering much more to my needs and towards my overall goal.

5. PERSONAL TRAINER: Getting external help for best results

Here's a thought: why do successful companies still have consultants there every week? Are they on the decline already and try all means to not go bankrupt? Or are they instead adapting to current market changes and rely on an exterior view on their processes and strategies, which they wouldn't see themselves by 'looking in the mirror'?

I made the same approach after I finished my first bunch of regular gym sessions. I could look into the mirror from some of the workout equipment, or could watch how fitness idols did their workouts in their videos and stories. But I realised that I am always open to **making slight mistakes** that could eventually **add up to doing it completely wrong** - and thus doing more harm than well in the worst case, throwing me back quite a few steps in the best case.

I therefore decided that it was better for my overall goal (and budget) to get external help every now and then in order to **get a professional and honest feedback** on how I do my workouts. Something a gym buddy is likely to oversee if he/she doesn't know better himself/herself, or doesn't want to risk ruining your feelings. It does have its costs to book half an hour or an hour of personal training - but if wrong workouts would put me off plan, resulting in say half a year longer to reach my goal, the personal trainings were a better investment for me in the long sight.

In retrospect I must admit that this had been the right decision for me: I got corrected early enough before falling into bad routines, and I got regular in-depth in-body analyses of my progress in important indices, like my muscle weight percentage, my body mass index (BMI) and my body fat percentage. **On top of all, it helped increase my motivation and dedication levels enormously.** And it stayed an important part of my healthy lifestyle as I wanted to strive for best results, not just average ones.

5 Learnings from this chapter:

1. Professional and honest feedback will avoid mistakes in your workouts.

2. Buddies can oversee such things, the pros shouldn't.

3. Personal trainings kept me on track with my progress.

4. Regular body index analysis kept me motivated and dedicated.

5. Personal trainers can become your 'professional buddies' for all their expertise.

6. TRACKING CALORIES: Awareness of what I actually eat

Whether it was counting points (with which I started out in the early days) or adding up calories (what I stuck to afterwards and still do), in order to incorporate a diet into my life I first had to become fully aware of what I actually eat in my life. Of what my habits were. What meal sizes I ate. And if the food mix throughout the day was something I'd be recommended to change by a nutritionist or a personal trainer, or if all was well already.

You might guess it already: **I was NOT fully aware of my eating and nutrition habits.** Although I studied a lot about it during my chef apprenticeship, although I was in the basketball team and cycled everywhere in town on my bike, I should have been more aware I thought at first. But those days were during my adolescence where my metabolism was not that of a grown adult yet, where working days and job life had just started, where I lived in an urban small town compared to a huge city nowadays.

I had heard of the concept that average men should eat approx. 2500 kcal per day, as a rough number, with women a bit less. But hey, looking around me every guy was different, so 2500 calories couldn't have been the exact number for me, could they? **I was curious of my own calorie input** and if it were at average or not at all - and so I started tracking my intake regularly.

The first hurdle I had to overcome was getting aware of food industry intentions, which healthy advertising was true and which was misleading me. Finding food products in supermarket aisles that were ‚low fat' or ‚fat free' mostly were true in marketing terms. Lower fat or less fat than the original product sometimes differed from my expectations - 2.4 grams of fat in light cheese versus 4.8 in the normal version was what I was looking for (equals -50 % fat and -30 % kcal). Less fat but MORE calories than the original, that was something I didn't think of finding but had to learn about very quickly. If less fat meant more sugar - believe me there are products out there in the supermarkets - then **it was time to look much closer at the ingredients and nutritional facts** printed on the labels. If the supposedly ‚more healthy' product was more expensive than the original on top of all, it was about time to rethink my shopping and eating habits even more, I realised.

It would result in quite longer shopping trips, maybe standing in the way of other customers while reading labels and comparing products - rather than just putting them into the shopping cart and off to the next aisle ... **but it had to be worth it for me!**

While tracking the calories of each food or snack I ate or drank, I slowly became aware that not all the stuff was really needed by my body. That there was some food I could have reduced or skipped after all. That was sometimes eaten not because of hunger but of pure pleasure, sometimes of previous conditioning.

Let's look at breakfast: when having moved to Munich I found the best tasting Pretzels so far. I loved eating a warm Pretzel freshly from the bakery's oven, and I went to buy one every day before work. I soon upgraded to the famous ‚Butter Pretzel' (sliced in half, spread with butter and garnished with chives). Wanna know the calorie intake straight away? Pretzel = 300 kcal (100 grams) and Butter Pretzel = 360 kcal. Okay, that's only 15 % of a 2500 kcal daily limit, but then again: 15 %? What would that leave throughout the rest of my day? **What would be lower calorie alternatives?** I wanted to find that out.

Lunchtime came next: and I literally mean next as in often just shortly after. My routine was an 08:00-09:00 a.m. start in the office, with an 11:30 a.m. mutual canteen lunch with my colleagues. After all, this next big meal of the day sometimes came only 2.5 hours after breakfast. It was a ritual at that time of day, but many times I did not _really_ feel hungry again. Leaving out this time with my colleagues completely was no longtime solution for me, as it is a valuable break time where you get to know you co-workers more privately and can switch off by having non work-related topics to talk about.

Tracking my food intake at lunch made me eat smaller sized portions after a while, portions up to the _level of my real hunger_. In the long run it made me shift the mix on my plate to 1/2 sizes of the main dish together with 1/2 the plate from the salad bar. As an example: Spaghetti Bolognese with Parmesan cheese = 430 kcal (250 grams) – roughly 20 % of the day's limit. – A 1/2 portion of the pasta and 1/2 a small mixed salad usually adds to about 285 kcal only (also 250 grams total weight), which is a third less calories.

But that wasn't usually it, can you relate to it? Canteens serve desserts as well, or I had bought yourself an item at the bakery earlier, when purchasing that Pretzel. A glazed donut (260 kcal), a chocolate muffin (300 kcal) or a French croissant (360 kcal) would fill my day's account with an easily unrecognised 10-15 % more – lunchtime over and my calories had already reached between 1000-1100, and I hadn't calculated any cappuccinos (80-100 kcal each) or smoothies (125 kcal per bottle) yet, which would easily leave me at 1500 kcal with an honest count.

And what about the afternoon? Eating some anti-stress chocolate or other office sweets later on were usual habits - or kind of 'automatic habits'- for me …

To make a long day short now: add buying take-out Indian tikka, salami pizza or a burger menu for dinner, and the additional calories (approx. 400, 800 or 900 kcal) brought me to an **average of 3000-3500 calories at the end of a day** - including the usual potato chips, salted peanuts and other evening snacks that I found in the kitchen cupboards. That was 20-40 % <u>more</u> of what should be enough for a man.

Was that one of the reasons why I grew more and more uncomfortable in my wardrobe? It was time for me to find out exactly what my own recommended calorie intake was, if the 2500 kcal were correct for me or not. And **using a health app helped me** rather easily and at no (or comparably low) costs.

Of course it takes time to weigh or roughly scale the different food items, enter them into the app, and not forget it at all. But what is 1 minute after each main meal, is it really such a long time? You could do that on the elevator, be honest. And the app can assist you with a barcode scanner or suggesting recently used items, so you'll get faster over time. If you change your mindset to this tracking process, it won't feel like wasted time anymore - but rather invested time, an investment into your healthy lifestyle.

Wanna compare my previous average days to how I eat now? Have a look:

My typical day then:

Breakfast:

Orange Juice 180 kcal

2 Coffee with milk 60 kcal

2 spoons of sugar 40 kcal

Butter Pretzel 360 kcal

Lunch & Afternoon:

Steak with potatoes 410 kcal

Gravy with cream 100 kcal

Apple Juice 180 kcal

2 Coffee with milk 60 kcal

Cappuccino 80 kcal

3 spoons of sugar 60 kcal

10 pieces of sweets 320 kcal

Dinner & Snacks:

Meat balls 400 kcal

Potato salad 200 kcal

4 pieces of cheese 250 kcal

Salted peanuts 600 kcal

Total: 3300 kcal (vs. 2300 kcal need)

<u>**My typical day now:**</u>

Breakfast:

Banana 100 kcal

Whey protein drink with milk 215 kcal

1 Coffee with milk 30 kcal

Coffee black 5 kcal

Sweetener instead of sugar 0 kcal

Lunch & Afternoon:

Steak with little bit of sauce 175 kcal

Mixed salads with dressing 125 kcal

1 Coffee with milk 30 kcal

Coffee black 5 kcal

Cappuccino 80 kcal

Dinner & Snacks:

Chicken 280 kcal

Vegetables 50 kcal

Asian sauces 50 kcal

Almonds 180 kcal

Conjac glass noodles 20 kcal

2 pieces of light cheese 80 kcal

Carrots 40 kcal

Pomelo 30 kcal

Whey protein drink with milk 215 kcal

Total: 1800 kcal (vs. 2300 kcal need)

<u>Remember:</u> this only reflects some of <u>my own</u> eating habits to illustrate what changes I underwent in the process. My 2300 kcal daily need as well as the food I ate are <u>not</u> blueprints for the perfect diet for you to copy!

Being aware of the impact my food intake had throughout the day, and how much spare calories I had left for use for small cheat food portions or carb side dishes - that was one of the great gains in my process of becoming a new me.

5 Learnings from this chapter:

1. Being aware of what I ate was a huge basis for my transformation.

2. Comparing nutritional facts will sort out the "fake healthy" from the healthy products.

3. Reducing the calorie food intake has a lot to do with changing the habits.

4. Tracking with a health app was the key to my progress.

5. Investing into the tracking time was an investment in me.

7. NUTRITION COACHING: Getting external dieting motivation

Over time I got much more aware of how much food or which food mix was helping my dieting process. What knowledge I was missing out on, though, became clearer when I was getting deeper looks into my tracking app via outside persons. When I got my macro nutrients mix adjusted to my current workout plan. When my food intake got analysed and I was given recommendations on how I could supplement some items with lower calorie alternatives or higher protein ingredients.

The first step was getting a change in my macro mix: my workout plan was aimed at increasing muscles and thus loosing body fat, so I learned that muscles recover and build up faster if a certain amount of proteins were eaten. My mix of 40 % carbs + 33 % proteins + 27 % fat (based on the grams intake and automatically set up through the app, within a "low carb" plan) got adjusted to 40 % carbs + 40 % proteins + 20 % fat. The calorie intake stayed identical, but the focus shifted to more protein and less fat.

What looked good straight away in the tracking app was a bit of a challenge in real life, however. I knew I could buy protein in bulk containers - lots of adverts appeared in my social media feeds by now - but for me that was stuff for the pros, for bodybuilders, for those who did competitions. But me? Just wanting to loose weight and get a bit more defined muscles? How could I eat so much proteins a day while having fun eating it? **For all I knew:** a chicken egg (medium size) has 7 grams of protein, my new daily goal was 140 grams, so in my head I compared the goal with eating 20 eggs each day, day in, day out. That sounded extremely dull and not fun! And changing 20 eggs to just powder drinks did not sound any better either. There had to be other foods that the fitness family ate, but somehow my mind had a blocking and always thought of the 20 eggs first.

‚**Ask the pro directly'** was the solution I said to myself! What had I to loose? So the next time I had a personal training I asked my coach directly WHAT HE ATE to reach his protein goal - and hoped it weren't eggs, egg-white scrambled eggs or whey powder as such. 😔 Real feedback was what I would believe more from than from theoretical stuff, 'cos the coach couldn't lie so much then. Dressed in sports clothes he couldn't hide his own results or progress - unless he was in a mass phase with the intention of gaining weight, which would be opposed to my phase. But still it were real feedback, face to face, eye to eye ... you're less likely to blankly lie in such situations, right?

And there I got my answers, straight from the professional, all real and personal nutrition advices like „After work I like to cook a **chicken breast** with a small salad and **cottage cheese**" or „I always have **skyr** in the fridge …". By these first hand infos I realised my mind started unblocking already and opening up. Cottage cheese I had known already, but **I was curious for skyr**.

With both of these however I realised I found new tasty food that contains enormously more protein than eggs: a small pot of cottage cheese (200 grams) has 24 grams of proteins, half a pot of natural skyr (250 grams) has 27 grams. That were the equivalents of 3-4 eggs or 3-4 portions (250 gram portions) of low fat yoghurt. Skyr was so much better than yoghurt - who would eat a kilo of yoghurt anyway, I realised quickly? Integrating these two into a day (e.g. skyr for breakfast and cottage cheese as an afternoon snack) would already account for almost 50 out of my 140 grams protein goal, and **it thus reduced the initial ‚protein hurdle' a lot** in order to reach the daily goal.

A few weeks into it I was proud of having many recommended protein foods on my shopping list regularly, and that I actually enjoyed eating them because I liked their taste. **But my coach still corrected me at this point**, he wanted me to FULLY open up and **see the full potential**. Why? Because my focus was on staying within my overall calorie limit, but <u>by not exceeding my carb limit</u> as first priority. When wanting best results for my muscles I needed to **shift my priority to filling up my proteins first** while keeping the overall limit in view. It was quite a big change in mindset for me, but after a while I realised it was possible to incorporate it into my diet. I made my personal campaign slogans as ‚PROTEINS FIRST' and ‚YES I CAN' to visualise and constantly remind me on the way. And with this new focus I started **finding more high protein foods** in the supermarket as well as in my lunch canteen:

- The supermarket started to offer quite a variety I ignored before, but when I made it a habit of taking a closer look at the nutrition labels, I found many new tasty foods to put on my plate.

- And in the canteen I found items I could combine, eat more of, or give feedback to the chefs to be put on a wish list - while still having a full and varied plate to eat for lunch, not thinking of losing out on anything or getting hungry too soon afterwards.

Opening up to **my ‚proteins first campaign'** I found myself saving more and more recipes that inspired me on social media. Posts and stories of interesting high protein recipes got screenshot and added in a new photo album on my phone. And when planning the shopping list for the next days or the weekend, I swiped through these inspirations to try myself. Such first hand meal stories by people from the fitness family inspired me more than nutritional theory books did - but I was still on my journey, and who says that things have to stay how they are.

After a while this rather personal look at some of my fitness role models made me take another step in my progress: **I signed up for a professional nutrition coaching** as a kind of upgrade to my current lifestyle. Why? I wanted to get daily direct feedback on my food intake while it was still fresh in my mind; on how I could adjust and do better every day; how I could make small changes before they'd manifest into a wrong habit; how I could supplement some foods with lower calorie alternatives; how these could be replaced by others if they didn't taste so well to me; and that I could get personalised recipes based on my taste (and my food allergies).

I must admit that those weeks (in July 2019) were some of the most challenging and also most focused ones so far. But I ended up reaching new interim goals, in my case without starving and with lots of fun and food variety. They were really rewarding to me when I took a look at my body indices, **what I was able to achieve!** This professional coaching lay the basis for all my future focus phases, as I knew I still wanted to progress. And that I would have to overcome times of being not so successful, times without progress.

So, which new food items do I still regularly incorporate into my diet these days?

- Conjac glass noodles (low carb),
- Chickpeas and lentils,
- Cottage cheese,
- Ice cream with protein,
- Protein whey powder shakes,
- Skyr,
- Tuna in water,
- Zoodles (low carb zucchini noodles).

5 Learnings from this chapter:

1. Being aware of what my food consists was another huge basis for my transformation.
2. Campaigning for 'Proteins First' helped me focussing.
3. Replacing food items isn't so hard, but professionals can lead you onto that track.
4. Being open to new food will change your diet in the long run.
5. Trust and ask the pros, that's what they're there for.

8. KEEP THE FUN: Learn how to progress even with pizza & co.

Many diets fail or are stopped early because food we are used to is restricted or completely forbidden. If it is food I remember and love since childhood days it's even harder for me to ban it from my grocery list. Try to think of food you really get a craving for - mine are e.g. licorice, pralinés, french fries and Gouda cheese. I can easily eat much more than I should, mostly because my brain saved some eating habits from when I was growing up - but let's be honest, my body needed much more calories when I was adolescent 'cos I still grew and transformed into an adult. **But after all, they were habits I still had as an adult.** If they were tiny portions or mini sizes of the original chocolate bars, then I could easily eat more than the equivalent normal bar size by far. Or when finding a complete corner piece of cheese in the fridge (that's how it is often sold in German supermarkets) I was tempted to eating at least half of that cheese block (250 grams) just like that, with nothing else aside. (Okay, maybe with mustard, I confess.)

With today's changed metabolism **I needed to train my body a different approach**: small doses of the food cravings would still satisfy my ‚sweet tooth' or ‚urge for savory' - that was the idea that grew in my head, that needed to manifest itself over time. It was not meant to strictly be a „just half diet" for everything or every plate I ate; I wanted to apply this concept particularly to those ‚nasty' carbs and sugars that were kinda sitting on my one shoulder together with that tiny devil, who kept repeating „eat it all, come on, you deserve it all for yourself".

Did I really have to eat it all by myself? Or could a **‚sharing is caring' approach** help me in keeping the fun in dieting, remaining friends with pizza, burgers, french fries and co? Let me practically show you how I implemented it, either when eating on my own or when having dinner the two of us:

- 1 Small salad + chicken nuggets **vs**. 1 full Burger menu including fries,

- Small pizza + carrot and cucumber sticks and a dip **vs**. Medium/large pizza + nothing,

- 1/2 a Medium pizza + a small salad each **vs**. 1 Medium/large pizza for each of us,

- 1/2 a Burger Menu including wedges (burger cut in half with knife) **vs**. 1 full menu,

- Just a piece of cheese (the rest put back in fridge) **vs**. The whole cheese on the table,

- Only a portion of potato crisps **vs**. The whole stack of crisps,

- Peanuts poured into a small bowl **vs**. Taking the original peanut container on the sofa.

Did I do something impossible here? Was slicing a burger in half a thing I shouldn't do?
Were I going too far? Or were I on the right track, on the way towards a better mindset
already? Was this a necessary next step within my progress? One that kept me going,
kept me having fun while doing this, kept me on track towards my goal?

I never said it was easy, and I can tell you how much I did long for much more bigger
portions, for just finishing it all in one go, believe me! But even if I could restrict myself
to only eating the so-called ‚cheat meals' once a week – I rather wanted to eat them
more than just one out of seven days, I wanted to enjoy them as regular ‚treat meals'
instead.

The biggest hurdle I often faced though was me tempting on giving up: „This one pizza
won't ruin my diet" … „This one super-sized burger menu won't do harm to my progress"
… „This chicken tikka masala with basmati rice will be fine – the rest of the week I'll eat
healthy" … „Okay from tomorrow I'll eat healthy" … „Alright, it's Friday night, the
weekend will be diet weekend" … Can you imagine how quickly the new routine I
started fell back into that old routine? The one where I was not conscious of what I ate,
how much I consumed, and what impact that lifestyle had? The one against which I had
made a contract with myself earlier, the contract I wasn't allowed to cancel early.

My new eating habits were different and hard to adjust to, I admit. They required
constant and consistent discipline from me. I really was my biggest enemy here!
But they kept the fun for me - without sacrificing completely on pizza & co.

5 Learnings from this chapter:

1. No food should be banned or completely forbidden.

2. Small sizes of your favourite cravings are okay.

3. One pizza alone won't ruin your diet – one per day is something different.

4. Make them small-sized treat meals, not complete cheat meals.

5. No huge cravings means no extreme jojo effect later.

9. HASHTAGS: Finding and creating your motivation

Hashtags for me aren't only for getting my posts and stories found on Insta or Facebook, moreover they are **a small dosis of motivation** by which I can express myself and my current focus. And also remind me consistently of what small goals make up for that big overall goal.

Here's my (never complete and always evolving) list of hashtags, saved in my notes app for quick use and reference:

#becauseitmattersforwhoyouredoingit

#bestversionofme

#betterthanyesterday

#discipline

#diffucultroadsleadtobeautifuldestinations

#dontstopuntilyoureproud

#fitfam

#getinshape

#goodvibes

#healthylifestyle

#justdoit

#knowyoucan

#makeyourselfapriority

#mindset

#motivation

#motivateyourself

#noexcuses

#onlywantingisntenough

#sticktoit

#stopwishingstartdoing

#summerbodiesaremadeinwinter

#teamfit

#twodaysinarow

#workingonanewme

5 Learnings from this chapter:

1. Motivate yourself by favourite expressions that inspire you.

2. Use inspirational words and phrases to motivate others on social media.

3. Subscribe to hashtags to connect to people with same interests.

4. Repeating words and phrases can help you focus better.

5. Encouraging phrases are a reminder of the small goals towards your overall goal.

10. SPREAD THE WORD: Tell others about your results

Communication coaches will tell you this, and you might have experienced it in the office as well: **do well and talk about it**, and you'll be likely to get more recognition, more interaction and more appreciation from your colleagues and your superiors.

During my fitness journey that was exactly what I wanted to get, in order to keep me going. I needed a bit of „well done" after a training, or a motivational 💪, 💯 or 🙌 as **virtual support** by followers. Not each and every time - remember I wasn't gonna turn into a full-time fitness model - but I also didn't want it to be unnoticed.

An easy item **to get recognised "offline"** was the sports bag: if you bring it to work (and you previously had no laptop bag, messenger bag or anything in your hands) you're sure to get noticed. Some will interact and ask if you're going to the gym after work, some will even ask since when you're doing sports ... and of course, you could easily also bump into a client on the way to the office building nearby, also carrying a sports bag. And this interacting into a small talk about sports on one day could help finding a mutual topic during the next coffee break, canteen lunch or client meeting. Or it might even lead to the founding on new running groups, registrations to business run events, or a corporate health movement start within the company.

When was the last time you gave somebody a genuine compliment? And how did you feel afterwards yourself? Did it boost your own positivity as well? Did it uplift your own day, too? Was your compliment contagious and you received a genuine one in return? **Appreciation gets and keeps you motivated - it can create a mindset that will make you succeed more easily.**

5 Learnings from this chapter:

1. Don't hide with your results, mini goals reached or success stories.

2. Appreciation will get you motivated, even virtually from strangers.

3. Giving genuine compliments to others can result in motivating responses.

4. Offline interaction on mutual sport topics can spark a variety of outcomes.

5. Do well and talk about it if you want your efforts to get recognised.

11. GO THE EXTRA MILE: Let your results be used against you

I am a person who likes talking and conversations, so during a one-hour personal fitness training I also need to do a bit of small talk. And like I do with my co-workers and clients, I don't hide some of my personal experiences from my trainer as well. These include positive experiences like (mini) goals reached, bad habits I wanted to break but still haven't, as well as habits I changed or new things I started.

What if your trainer wants you to do a bit more than usual, always exceed your limits by just a bit more - knowing you'll make it and it won't hurt you much? Well, he's/she's **making you go the extra mile**. So if you're really proud of something you achieved or changed, he/she will acknowledge this and praise you, of course - and afterwards will **use your achievement against you**! To show you that there's even more potential in you, and that you can easily go that extra mile!

The thing is: YOU KNOW YOU CAN! 😉

You already made an effort to be better than yesterday, that means you're very likely willing to make that special effort to really achieve your goal. If you know that you can do more than what is expected, why wait for it? Train a little harder, go above the norm or act outside the box. Make more progress and grow beyond your initial goals. Difficult roads lead to beautiful destinations - and guess what: they're usually never crowded.

If you want to become the best version of yourself, stop wishing and start doing.

For me personally that meant a "challenge accepted" approach and mindset, and kind of seeing the progress like a multi-level computer game:

- Keeping on sharing my proud moments with my personal trainer, no matter what.

- Not fearing constructive feedback with corrective measures at the end of it.

- A good performance could always be levelled up to a great performance.

- Growing from a "great" performer to "the best" was completely up to myself.

- If Level 1 was finished easily, my hard work determined how quickly level 2 ended.

Wanna know some of my proud-moments-turned-into-new-challenges?

- I'm one of a few that walks down 12 storeys by stairway from the office to the canteen or the client appointment. **–>** Why not start walking UP the stairs as of tomorrow? You won't need a stairs trainer in the gym anymore!

- Do you know how exhausting 12 storeys upstairs are? **–>** Why not start with 3 storeys by stairs and the rest by elevator? And gradually add more storeys over time, until you're fit for all twelve?

- Hey, I am eating less sugar and more protein already! **–>** So why are you buying a brand product protein chocolate pudding from the supermarket that has lots of added protein - yes - BUT almost as much sugar as the brand's original chocolate pudding?

- Okay, I'm not often eating that brand protein pudding anymore! **–>** Why don't you drastically reduce your consumption of ANY convenience food, take-out meals and delivery dinners?

- After last time's 6:00 a.m. personal training I was much more focused in the office and took less/almost no time to 'boot up my system'! **–>** Why not make it a habit to hit the gym 3 times a week at early bird hours? Even if it's just for 30-45 minutes?

You could add a 'hmmm ...' 😐 after each of the above - and probably have similar examples from your own personal experience at hand, am I right? Did these advices make you feel motivated afterwards? Did you want to show that person that you definitely can do that, too? "**Now more than ever!**"? Then you've already got what it takes! Keep on rolling, get into motion and get the momentum going!

5 Learnings from this chapter:

1. Be proud of your achievement and accept additional challenges immediately after.

2. Don't be afraid of going the extra mile.

3. Seek the fun in any new challenge - new trainings ideas & habits might be the result.

4. Stop wishing to become the best version of yourself - start doing it.

5. Show the world that you can make it! Now more than ever!

12. DAILY DOSE: Small routines lead to faster progress

Finding daily routines is the key to becoming successful in many areas and aspects. Can you relate to this: often you find yourself planning on doing something, but later put it off because it will take too long, is too big a project or it's too late and you're too tired already.

Breaking bigger tasks down into many small tasks will make the tasks easier to finish, you'll feel successful more often and keep motivated to sticking to it. Staying on track will thus lead to a faster progress, as the sum of the many small steps you reached is already bigger than the one-time big step you planned to do initially.

Try to remember the last time you wanted to start with something - quit smoking, eat healthier, do more sports, call friends & family regularly - and how long you postponed this resolution or quit it completely.

Over time I have extended the daily dose approach - or setting mini goals and reaching them comparatively quick - to the following parts in my life throughout the day:

- Podcasts

- Financial newspapers

- Industry news

- Book summaries

- Keeping contact within professional networks

- Commenting posts/stories

- Writing down blog ideas and other notes (including when writing this book).

Why did I mention ‚throughout the day' earlier? Because the time for reaching my small goals is not only at the end of my working day. If your day doesn't start like a ‚rocket launch' when out of bed, **there'll be a few time slots each day** into which you can fit a few routines. Think about how long you take to finish your first coffee at home, and what could fit exactly in this time. Or what you could do while brushing your teeth, waiting at the bus stop, commuting to work, or walking downstairs to the canteen? These are just some examples that you could integrate before lunchtime. Same applies for when leaving the office or even when chilling in bed on a Sunday morning. Unless you're an extreme workaholic, you will find plenty of short spare times each day - believe me.

If you are a digital person, find yourself a smartphone app for support. This way you'll have it close at hand anytime since the phone is your most used device anyway. 😅 In order to stop procrastinating your routines, **shift all these apps onto your main screen**. This way you're more likely to be reminded by the app's logo whilst doing ‚normal' stuff like reading a message, checking your mails or doing app updates.

Did this small routine approach help me with my fitness goals as well, what do you guess? Of course it did, and it gave me self-motivation to keep progressing. How?

- Starting with 3 km runs, extending them to 4, 6, then 8 km before knowing I can easily register for the 10 km business run. And then finish my training course after 15 km when the exhaustion level was at my real max, exceeding my initial goal by far.

- Choosing 3 flights of staircases upwards and then taking the elevator to the 12th floor, gradually increasing by one flight after time. Until I made the 12 stories in one go and without needing a bed to rest afterwards.

- Tracking a calorie deficit of 300-500 kcal per day to progressively loose approx. 300-500 grams body weight per week - instead of wanting to reach an impossible minus 10 kilos in just a month, in 10 days or other typical dieting timeframes you usually come across in adverts or magazines.

I'm sure you're probably thinking of a few things already, that you can simply start as of tomorrow, am I right? 😎 Then go ahead and start doing them - **in fact: start today!**

Optional: Share your success stories or posts by tagging me (@hanjokoch).

5 Learnings from this chapter:

1. Break down your overall goal into a couple of mini goals.

2. Adding up many small steps isn't as hard as trying to make one huge step right away,

3. Determine short time slots throughout the day that you used differently before.

4. Accomplish mini goals in various parts of your life, in which you aim to progress.

5. Get digital support via apps, and keep them at sight on the main screen.

13. BREAK THE ROUTINE: Planning the daredevil

Did you ever/lately find yourself skipping gym because going there seemed boring all of a sudden? You know all the corners and devices by heart, and your workout playlists don't motivate you anymore? Each of us might come to a point like this sometime …

This is called routine – and you'll have come across it in various ways in your life already: same walk or ride to school over years, grocery shopping in the same supermarket, same car route for commuting to work, same cabin on the train or metro going home …

Well, what were your reactions to these when you got bored, **did you just give up**? Or did you walk a slightly different way, around another block? Buy your vegs and meat at the competitive brand, down the road. Drive the second fastest route recommended by the app or navigation system? Sit at the opposite end of the cabin or the train? If you already did this in such common life situations, why not apply it to your workouts as well?

If your gym is part of a brand with more than one outlet in your city, changing locations every now and then could help you. Even if you're doing identical workouts there, you'll find the machines in different areas due to the overall setup, you'll see different faces there, different trainers and customers. They might even have differing brands where adjusting the weights isn't the same way. **What does all that do with me during workouts?** From my experience I was more conscious in the new location, more aware of my surroundings, more concentrated during my workouts. And overall my motivation level didn't decline but rather stay put or sometimes even increased.

If your gym is stand-alone or your town has only this one gym, it's more difficult of course. But hey, you're not a robot after all, so still plenty of new options available for you.

Wanna know **what I did to break my routines**, how I turned upcoming de-motivation into motivation? How I planned on being a daredevil against life's routines? Here's a few:

- Time of day: join the ,06:00 a.m. club' with a pre-office workout in the morning, or skipping Sunday breakfast in lieu of an early gym session.

- Day of the week: postpone the regular Saturday morning grocery shopping into the afternoon and do your sports in that time slot.

HANJO KOCH   Working on a new me

- Change location: go to a different gym branch every few workouts, or sign up for two cheap gyms that won't cost more than one medium priced contract.

- Add disciplines: if you enjoy swimming, running, cycling or badminton – add these in between your gym trainings to bring variety into your sports life.

- Make daily spare time: get up just 15 minutes earlier than usually and use them for home bodyweight exercises like sit-ups, squats, push-ups, bridges or elbow planks.

- Use daily spare time: TV commercial breaks can vary between 3 to 9 minutes during prime time, why not do short exercises during these intervals?

- Find gym devices in everyday situations: why wait for the stair climber at the gym when you can take stairs up to your apartment or office?

- Reach 10.000 steps per day: enter the tram or metro one stop later than usual, or park the car on a farther parking space than the closest one.

- Don't find excuses: bring your gym bag to work and leave it there, so you can't find an excuse that you first have to go home – you've already got what it takes to work out.

- Think outside the box: bring your running gear to work and run (a part of your journey) home; the next day bring a bag to take home yesterday's office clothes.

- Every little helps: find a solution for bits of exercises as often as possible, this way you can reach and exceed the general goal of 30 minutes of moderate physical activity.

Was this inspiring enough? **The above were true examples** with which I broke the chains of many of my previous routines. It meant changing my mindset in some cases, overcoming my inner barriers and spending a bit more time than before. But unless your spare time is non-existent there'll be ways for you to incorporate a similar healthy lifestyle, and a lot of times without a major cash investment at all.

5 Learnings from this chapter:

1. Recognise the routines in your life.

2. Find easy to apply solutions by changes in timing, locations or habits.

3. Add variety to increase your sports motivation.

4. Think outside the box when feeling stuck or uncreative.

5. Be a daredevil and plan ahead to break your routines.

14. SIDE EFFECTS: How my job got affected

Privately focussing on goals and habits automatically had an influence into my professional life as well, though mostly unintentionally in the beginning. Over time I gradually realised that some things I learned at the gym could be adapted to my job - affecting my performance positively.

What behaviours made me more focussed then? How did my office routines change. My first order was: **The past, regardless of what it has been so far, is in the past.** My second order was: **The future is flexible, the future is now. So concentrate on it!**

Show up a little earlier: If I could get some exercises done by getting out of bed 15 minutes earlier than before, I could also get some things done when sitting at my desk a bit earlier than usual. I started having some 'secret minutes' to myself, where colleagues were mostly unaware of me being available already. And I spent the time catching up on management reports and previous day statistics, brainstorming on creative input needed or simply getting my day organised.

Invest more in myself: The early office time was also reserved for a learning ritual: reading the industry newsletters to stay up to date on trends and news daily. To be able to react if key account companies were involved or affected, if topics we to be found in their press releases as well, and a personal call to my contract person should be on my agenda. In today's changing environment of shareholder value news, mergers or acquisitions it is valuable to stay updated.

Write down my 3 top to-dos, every single morning: Handwriting down or digitally organising my three most important to-dos was based on the concept of signing a contract with myself. Knowing I had to finish these three tasks by end of day, no matter what, I had set myself an internal deadline - without the external pressure by others. And if unexpected urgent tasks came up during the day, it wasn't impossible to finish these three cases without putting them into overtime hours.

Prioritise my top 3 as first things first: I made my top 3 to-dos my priority to finish before the first management meeting - in my case the daily 10:00 a.m. operations meeting. The similarities to my sports life were like the main gym session workouts I wanted to include, even during the prime time when the gym was crowded.

Eliminate all non-priorities: Although I liked my cardio workout a lot in the beginning, I realised that jogging and the like had to become a non-priority, compared to the muscle buildup focus through weight lifting. In the office I learned to say "no" more often to requests and opportunities without scalable monetary outcome: if it won't influence a customers' request, can it be postponed to later in the afternoon? If I can reach customers by phone in the morning, ask to postpone an internal meeting request to a time slot where customers are usually harder to reach: over lunch hours or in afternoon.

Fast from the mailbox for 2 hours, twice per day: When in the gym or jogging, I do not answer phone calls at all. My phone gives me access to music playlists, audio books and podcasts - but also social media and other distractions. During sports hours I focus on the sport solely. I concentrate on achieving the best workouts, with correct posture and effective weights. I started doing a similar approach in the office: I blocked four hours daily for concentrated tasks, two hours before and two after lunch. My 'focus hours' are those where I plan not to get distracted, where I even put my company mobile phone on silent mode, when I switch off the 'new mail notifications' or the mail program completely. I'll get the occasional call by a colleague referring to a mail you therefore never heard of nor teaser-read at all - but you'll also realise that some things will have already been solved by then or by somebody else who was available earlier than you. And sometimes you weren't the top specialist for that issue, so moving those mails straight into a folder won't do any harm.

Focus on day-sprints rather than a month's marathon: By sticking to finishing 3 top to-dos per day, the results were visible to me very clearly every day. Trying to finish a huge workload of stuff that I postponed needed much more time in the end, as I couldn't scale it properly in advance, and it usually incurred in a lot of overtime hours - overall feeling more like an exhausting marathon run. The comparison to jogging was a simple one I could easily grasp, because I would not have tried waiting a month with no sports and then running a marathon from scratch instead.

Finish something unpleasant everyday that I procrastinated: In the gym it was usually my personal trainer that asked me which workout I did NOT want to do in today's training, or which exercise I hated - and then purposely had me do exactly that exercise a few minutes later. The outcome: overall I felt better after finishing this exercise, and I'm still alive ... so it couldn't have been that hard. 😄 Same applies in the job for unpleasant stuff that's not on my priority to-do list. If it's not urgent and not bringing in much revenue, I postpone it usually for a while. Finishing one per day won't leave me with a full day of doing just those tasks, which would leave me rather dissatisfied at the end of the day.

HANJO KOCH   Working on a new me

Walk and stand up A.M.A.P (as much as possible): When I first started gym exercises, my trainer told me quite frankly: "Let me guess, you have an office job with most time spent at your desk, correct?" From my posture he could easily tell, and of course he was damn right. 'But how could I change my habits in the office then?' I asked. Here were some easy steps at hand: Walk to the printer myself instead of waiting for a co-worker to bring my papers along; don't slide to the printer on my chair; walk to the colleague down the corridor instead of calling or emailing; stand up during a phone call; hold short operations meetings standing up; take the staircase downstairs on my way to lunch or on the way home; walk to the more distant public transport stop.

De-clutter the desk: Do I really need scissors, hole punch, 5 different pens and a stapler always at hand right in front of me on my desk? Or can they be put in a drawer, which wouldn't cost me five seconds more when taking them out only when needed? Removing all non-essentials from my desk got me much more organised and with a clearer mindset. The same applied at the gym: I didn't need to 'reserve' all areas in the gym that were part of my workout cycle. I only needed the vital basics with me at all times (towel, water bottle, headphones and smartphone for music) and then switched from exercise to exercise as the areas became free again.

Visualise my achievements: I have monthly goals of phone calls and personal client appointments to achieve, so-called KPIs (key performance indicators). Instead of counting them up at the end of the month, I checklist them on a sticky note, and add them every day. That way I see my progress over the course of each week, and can feel less stressed. Before hitting the gym regularly, I visualised my home cycling training by writing a logbook of the kilometres cycled - but as if I drove them on a motorway. That way I sketched a tour through Germany, and was really proud when finishing the round tour that brought me from Cologne to Hamburg, Berlin, Dresden, Munich, Stuttgart, Frankfurt and back home. I still do this when taking the stairs up to the 12th floor of the office by the way: if I do this only twice a day (e.g. before work and after lunch) I have already reached the top of Cologne Cathedral in my hometown (533 steps). If I do this 7 days in a row, I will have reached the top of the Empire State Building (1576 steps). Got my case? 😉

                          Working on a new me

Stop obsessing about a 100 % perfect outcome all the time: I don't need perfect weather conditions for an outdoor run. "Just do it" is the right motto here, if it looks like it might rain later I usually do a smaller round, so I won't have too much distance home if it does start raining. The outcome is still higher than if I didn't jog at all. Going to the gym for 30 minutes "only" is still better than not going at all. 😶 In the job I try to act by the 80-20 formula with allowing myself only 80 % perfection, saving the 20 % time for listening to others' opinions early in the project's process; or reinvesting the saved minutes into another project on my priority list. Or ticking off that "unpleasant" task I still had on my to-do list.

Focus on progress over time: Great things take time … that goes for reaching this year's revenue budgets as well as achieving my weight loss and muscle gain goals. Neither can happen in a day, a week or just like that. Each will need consistent efforts and repetition of proven processes. Constantly focussing on the goal is the key, that is what I realised.

Do what it takes and focus. Period. Hopefully enough said. 😐

So if you feel ready for some change, just look around … no one is stopping you!* 😏

* No one other than yourself.

5 Learnings from this chapter:

1. What I learned in sports could be adapted to my job as well.

2. Get up earlier to get things done.

3. Prioritise on 3 tasks to accomplish each day.

4. Also finish one unpleasant task per day, and thus work against procrastination.

5. Great things take time - so focus on the small "day-sprints" instead of the "marathon".

15. GYM B4 MEETING: What your posture and mindset do

Have you lately had an early morning business **meeting with the big boss, that you did not look forward to at all**? Because you remember how the last meeting turned out? And **how you felt during that previous meeting**? The one where the boss was really unhappy with the results, talked nearly all the time, didn't even find one positive feedback? And somewhat just ordered one new action plan after the other from you and everyone else in the meeting room? And all in all you felt rather small, downcast and frankly like s**t after this meeting?

So as soon as **you're invited to such a 9:00 a.m. meeting again**, you immediately remember how you felt after the last one and are thus bound to enter the meeting room with low hopes; you'll sit at the boardroom table looking down on your notes; and just **hope that this meeting will be over and done with soon**?

Well first of all, you can't blame your boss for the early morning timing: most people have the **highest energy level in the morning**/mid-morning. So if your superior wants the best interaction, discussions and problem solving from the team, no afternoons will likely be chosen to hold such meetings.

And secondly, you can't blame the boss for reacting to **what he sees upon entering the boardroom**. Why? Well, what exactly does he find there, be honest? In my example:

- a guy sitting in his chair but looking down instead of making eye contact,

- hunched over or slouching instead of sitting upright in the chair,

- seemingly unprepared instead of ready for an interaction with the boss.

And **your body language** sends this message to your colleagues as well as your boss:

- I don't really know what I'm doing here,

- I'm not confident in what I am doing,

- so don't expect me to be of valuable help for you during this meeting.

No wonder if your boss is picking on you with special attention and extra tasks - he/she is paying your monthly wages, and is expecting to get much more in return than an employee slouching around in the meeting room furniture. Fair enough, **you'd expect the same from your own team members**, am I right?

Whenever I had meetings coming up where I anticipated a similar scenario for me, from now on **I planned ahead**: a 09:00 a.m. meeting start meant 08:30 being in the office latest, half an hour commuting meant leaving around 08:00 o'clock. That left me with just the right amount of time to get up really early - **remember the ‚06:00 a.m. club'** - and start my morning with a pre-office workout. Or in this case a pre-meeting workout.

The **effects** that this triggered **on my mindset** were somewhat unexpected for me:

- I had suffered (muscle) pain and exhaustion already **–>** today can't get any worse;

- I've mastered heavy weights today already **–>** new tasks won't be a burden today;

- If you just got up (shortly before the meeting) with the wrong foot and are still grumpy **–>** well, my day is going to be great, and I won't let you get me down!

Effects on my posture and my **body language**:

- Sitting upright in my chair **–>** first impression will be that I belong here;

- Automatically looking up and making eye contact **–>** I am confident, boss;

- Getting up with quicker motion for a handshake **–>** I am of valuable help for you.

The most important outcome for me: meetings I usually anticipated to be bad ones turned out to be **productive meetings**, with **interaction** between the boss and us, with **discussions** and different points of views, with **praise** for tasks well done, **constructive feedback** with room for improvements - and most of all, the rest of the workday still ahead with **satisfaction and motivation instead of frustration**.

And seeing it from my boss' perspective: if meeting one was productive, entering meeting two with an overall positive mindset will have an enormous influence on how following meetings will start and their outcome - how the day for the whole team will be. **My sports could trigger a positive chain reaction for my co-workers** - even if it were just a small out of many sparks.

5 Learnings from this chapter:

1. Hitting the gym before a meeting will positively change your mindset and posture.

2. Sitting (and standing) straight with relaxed shoulders shows positive body language.

3. Good posture will increase your self-confidence and leave a better first impression.

4. Productive meetings will result in higher satisfaction and motivation levels.

5. Your sports can trigger a positive chain reaction for your co-workers.

Learnings from my own progress:

Now should have been the end of my written down experiences, a summary of what I learned over the past 2.5 years into my progress. **How I reached my fitness goal - and how a healthy lifestyle affected my job as well.** At least this was my plan, according to the schedule I had roughly planned ahead.

However, life as I knew was about to change quite drastically all of a sudden, and I had to adjust to it in many ways. The worldwide pandemic of the corona virus also forced me into a kind of lockdown, staying at home, with restriction of movement for only the most necessary things, social distancing, office tower closing and weeks of home office.

I therefore decided to **reflect on this new situation** and postpone finalising my summary - I wanted to see what impact would happen to my progress, both in positive or in negative results. If all I had achieved so far could be **a good basis to get me through this crisis** - and to come out stronger (or ideally not any weaker!).

Let me take you on this journey in the following bonus chapter.

16. BONUS: Impacts of the corona virus lockdown/home office

It was mid March 2020 when Germany got affected heavily by the corona virus (COVID-19) outbreak. Quite rapidly both my private and my job life were put into crisis mode and many restrictions applied suddenly. These weeks should have been the focus months where I concentrated on fine tuning muscle gains and weight loss towards my new second goal, according to my plan. And they should have been the weeks for fine tuning and finishing this book. Somewhat my plan seemed to be overruled by a higher power now that wanted me quitting all I had reached so far, that wanted me to accept the new circumstances of staying at home, that wanted my resignation.

What had changed all of a sudden? You will likely relate to this scenario:

- **Private interaction** was reduced to the minimum, meaning no spontaneous or unnecessary grocery shopping, no meeting friends for a coffee or an after work drink, nor going out for dinner to a restaurant, and no gym sessions anymore.

  - Instead: weekly shopping trips to reduce contacts and increase social distancing, phone calls or video chats with friends and family, and either jog alone outside or done home gym exercises for fitness.

  - My physical activity was much less due to lesser distances walked each day, apart from the cancelled fitness centre workouts.

- **Professional interaction** was moved from the office into home office, meaning no more team meetings, project meetings, on the job trainings, interaction with other departments down the corridor, canteen lunch breaks or coffee chats with co-workers, and no more client appointments which is the basis of my sales life.

  - Instead: setting up a home office, phone calls and video meetings, lunch and coffees on my own, and client appointments postponed for many weeks due to them being in identical situations as me.

  - Missing completely was the activity that commuting to and from work engaged, and along with that the distance you make when walking to a meeting, to an appointment, to another office, or to the canteen taking the stairs down 12 stories.

With this massive lack of activity in my life, images doomed to me of a guy who would fail after all, who gave up on all he had achieved so far, who accepted the excuse that the efforts were simply impossible due to the virus and the forced new lifestyle. Images of "me the couch potato", "me as the fat guy in the hover chair in the animated movie Wall-e", "me with two identical transformation photos where no change had happened".

I didn't want that to happen!

Now was the time to stick to my routines, focus on the essential learnings throughout my progress, keeping a positive mindset and making the best out of it.

It was time to shine!

Why were all this so important to me? Hard times bring up your real state of mind, they will show you how much you lie to yourself every day.

- When was the last time you told yourself "Today is the day!" - and then did nothing about it?

- Why always wait for the next opportunity? Don't wait for others to push you.

- Put in other words: the grass is greener at the point where you water it.

So instead of lying to myself, it was time to take action and adapt to change. With all the progress I had made so far, I had already designed my ideal day. I had found ways and concepts to maximise the amount of time I spend on my top priorities (both fitness and job wise). I had formed new habits of purposefully creating extra time every day to progress, improve and stay productive, for example by getting up 15 mins. earlier than before. Spare times were now times to skill up (with podcasts or financial news reading etc.). **Now phase 2 of living my dreams started: living my ideal day consistently.**

- The economy was in a recession and things were shutting down - but I didn't have to!

- A big hill was and still is going to be ahead in order to overcome this recession, in fact a monumental one. Monumental for all of us.

- Whatever I could do for my goals and my career - now was the time to get focused.

- Not to hide myself into distractions and my comfort zone.

- Don't hit pause on my dreams or my discipline.

- Prioritise NOW.

- Skill up NOW.

- Get disciplined NOW.

- Get moving and build a momentum in all my major projects.

- Don't wait for tomorrow for something I could have done today.

- My future self should always be proud of me and thank myself!

To live my ideal day, even though in crisis mode, I kept a daily routine like this one:

06:30 am: Alarm as usual, **no snooze button** allowed.

06:35 am: Start **45 mins.** home gym **exercises**, with workout variance on following day. Listen to news and motivational podcasts during sports, invest in myself part 1.

07:20 am: **Finish home gym**, drink a protein shake and check social media quickly.

07:30 am: Jump into shower. Shave and **get styled as on a usual working weekday**. Get dressed into business casual with a chino, t-shirt and basic pullover.

08:00 am: **"Commute" for 30 mins.** by walking through the apartment, reaching a first part of my walk-A.M.A.P.-goal. Listen to an approx. half-hour **podcast** or two "longer" fifteen minute podcasts. Vary with taking the stairs in the complex' corridors down & up.

08:30 am: Make myself a **small breakfast**, including coffee and large glass of water.

09:00 am: Open my work laptop and **start my home office** weekday. Prioritise on my **top 3 tasks** to be finished until midday.

10:00 am: Planned **5 mins. break for walking around**, making coffee or filling up water.

11:00 am: Planned 5 mins. **break** for walking around, filling up water glass.

12:00 pm: Planned lunch break. Prepare lunch and **eat at a different location** from the laptop desk. **Listen to radio or a playlist** via speakers to compensate missing co-workers in the canteen. Walk through apartment for 5-10 mins. to copy the usual walk back from the canteen. Vary with taking the stairs in the complex' corridors down & up.

12:30 pm: Back at the desk to continue home office. Don't forget **large glass of water**.

13:30 pm: Planned 5 mins. **break for walking around**, making coffee or filling up water.

14:30 pm: Planned **5 mins. break** for walking around, filling up water glass.

15:30 pm: Planned 15 mins. break for a **breath of fresh air** on the balcony, walking around, checking professional networks, making coffee or filling up water.

16:30 pm: Planned 5 mins. **break** for walking around, filling up water glass.

17:30 pm: End of workday, leave home office. **"Commute" for 30 mins.** by walking through the apartment, reaching **part two of my walking goal**. Listen to longer podcasts. Vary again with taking the stairs in the complex' corridors down & up.

18:00 pm: "Arrive at home", **change outfit** from business casual to comfy casual wear. Take time to **invest in myself** part 2 by reading a book summary.

18:30 pm: Start **normal after work evening** scenario with preparing dinner, social media, watching TV or videos, phone calls and such, followed by **bedtime routine**.

17. LEARNINGS FROM MY OWN PROGRESS

To sum up what this added *unplanned bonus time* made me realise, combined with the learnings during my progress over the past 2.5 years, here are my experiences & gains.

If I didn't come out of all of this with:

- **New skills** - while others just netflixed and procrastinated,

- **More knowledge** - by investments into myself,

- **More focus** - by setting up a binding self contract,

- **New workouts** - experiencing the advantages of weight lifting vs. cardio,

- **Higher dedication** - through the help of a personal trainer,

- **Better progress** - through regular body index analysis,

- **More awareness** - especially of my food intake and eating habits,

- **Full potential** - reached with nutritional coaching,

- **Having fun while dieting** - with small-sized treat meals,

- **New inspiration** - by following and using motivational hashtags,

- **Higher motivation** - personally or virtually from others,

- **New perspectives** - by allowing new challenges and breaking the routine,

- **New habits** - what helps in sports can be related to my professional office life,

- **Better results** - a change in mindset will impact sports and job progresses,

- **A life others still dream of** - while I took small steps regularly to reach my dreams,

... then I never lacked TIME before, in fact I lacked DISCIPLINE.

HANJO KOCH   Working on a new me

18. MY JOURNEY: See my indices in my timeline

I never said it was easy to reach my fitness goals, nor that it only took a few weeks. So I summarised some of my in-body analysis indices for you in this timeline. It has been a longer progress **with many small steps and in-between goals** achieved. Looking a the interim results regularly and relating them to what changes I had done in that period helped me understand my body and my habit changes much more.

For this chart I have selected my calorie deficit (if less than 100 %) and calorie surplus, body weight, muscle weight, body mass index and body fat percentage; over a time span of 29 months, with the detailed* outlines on the past 12 months.

** March 2020 figures missing and April 2020 figures that are identical to February could not be accurately tracked due to the fitness center closing whilst corona virus lockdown, therefore no access to official body analysis device.*

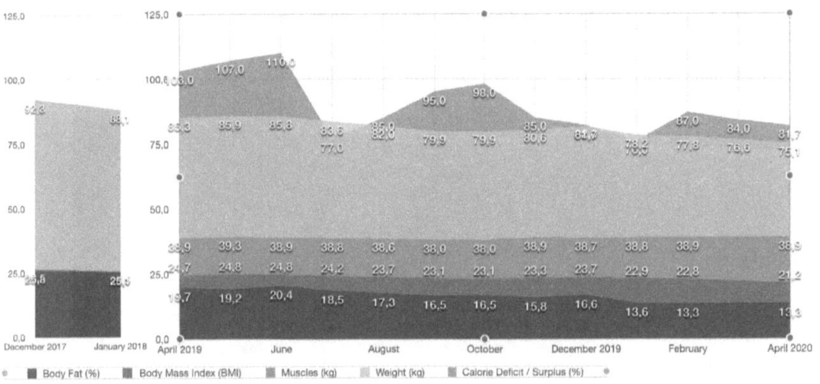

Remember: This is not explaining scientifically proven studies in detail, there is plenty of literature available in stores and libraries for that. It is intended solely as a motivational read for seeking inspiration, comparing results and progresses. This can vary for you depending on your own current circumstances, physique, mindset, lifestyle, workout intensity and more — so please don't see this chart as an ultimate blueprint.

19. RECIPES: My favourite food for inspiration

I want to share with you three recipes I have been cooking repeatedly over time, that I never got tired of cooking regularly. Give them a try yourself, adjust them according to your personal gusto, or use them as an inspiration to try out new ingredients you never bought before.

I've chosen a breakfast, a weekend lunch and a weeknight dinner for you.

Berry, avocado, cucumber and skyr breakfast smoothie (low sugar)

Fruit and vegetable smoothies with no added sugars are a quickly prepared breakfast alternative to bowls of cornflakes or muesli.

Total time: approx. 10 minutes   Prep time: 5 minutes   Cook time: 5 minutes

Calories: approx. 380 kcal per person   Servings: 1 portion   Cuisine: American

Ingredients:

- 75 g Berries like Strawberries, Blueberries and Raspberries

- 1 Kiwi fruit, without skin

- Half a lime, squeezed to juice

- 50 g Cucumber

- Half an Avocado fruit

- 50 g Skyr

- 100 ml Skimmed Milk (1.5 %)

Instructions:

1. Add all ingredients to a blender and blend (on high level) until creamy.

2. Make smoothie thinner by adding a bit of water.

3. Serve in a tall glass with a thick straw, or leave it in the portable travel cup.

Nutrition:

Calories: 380 kcal | Carbs: 26 g | Protein: 13 g | Fat: 20 g | approximately per person

Variations:

Use almond milk, Greek yoghurt, orange juice or carrot juice, and add banana, cinnamon powder, chia seeds or whey protein powder (might increase the thickness). Use half of the recipe when serving a thick smoothie along with a porridge & fresh fruit salad bowl.

Cottage cheese & mango salad with egg and roasted almonds (high protein)

This combination of sweet and savoury is packed with proteins and makes a light and healthy late-lunch option for the weekend.

<u>Total time</u>: approx. 15 minutes   <u>Prep time</u>: 5 minutes   <u>Cook time</u>: 10 minutes

<u>Calories</u>: approx. 320 kcal per person   <u>Servings</u>: 2 portions   <u>Cuisine</u>: Salad

Ingredients:

- 200 g Cottage Cheese, light

- 1 Mango, cut into cubes

- 2 Boiled Eggs, cut into four pieces

- 50 g Sweet Corn, drained

- 1 table spoon of Honey

- 20 g Roasted Almonds

- Fresh Chives, chopped

- Salt & Fresh Ground Pepper

Instructions:

1. Boil the eggs in a pot for 8-10 minutes until hard (as desired). Drain under cold water to cool down afterwards. Peel off the shell, cut into four pieces each, and set aside.

2. In the meantime add the almonds into a cold pan and turn to medium heat. Stir every few seconds until evenly roasted, careful not to burn them by forgetting to stir. Lightly salt as desired and leave set aside in the warm pan.

3. Toss the mango pieces together with the sweet corn, half of the chopped chives, honey and cottage cheese in a bowl and mix evenly.

4. Season with salt and fresh ground pepper as desired.

5. Serve in a bowl, garnish with the four pieces of egg, the (still warm) almonds and sprinkle with the remaining chives.

Nutrition:

Calories: 320 kcal | Carbs: 27 g | Protein: 22 g | Fat: 12 g | approximately per person

Variations:

Use agave syrup or maple syrup for sweetening, add cherry tomatoes, season with curry powder or chilli powder, or add rocket salad as a basis layer when serving on a plate.

Stir-fry Asian chicken with veggies and conjac glass noodles (low carb)

This low calorie version of a takeout favourite combines chicken, broccoli, bell pepper, ginger and conjac glass noodles for a delicious weeknight dinner.

Total time: approx. 30 minutes   Prep time: 20 minutes   Cook time: 10 minutes

Calories: approx. 335 kcal per person   Servings: 2 portions   Cuisine: Chinese

Ingredients:

- 2 chicken breasts, skinless, cut into slices

- 1 medium head of Broccoli, cut into florets

- 1 bell pepper, cut into cubes

- 2 pieces of spring onion, cut into small rings

- 1 inch piece of ginger, peeled and chopped

- 200 grams of Conjac glass noodles, drained under water

- 1 table spoon of vegetable oil

- 2 table spoons of soy sauce

- 2 table spoons of Sweet Chilli Asian sauce

- 4 table spoons of water

- 2 tea spoons of Sesame Seeds

- Fresh ground pepper as desired

Instructions:

1. Steam the broccoli florets to the desired softness & set aside.

2. Heat a pan or wok over a high heat and add the oil. Add the chicken and fry until brown and crispy on all sides. Remove from pan and set aside,

3. Fry the spring onion in the remaining oil in the pan, adding the ginger for 30 seconds. Add the bell pepper, tossing now and then until brown, letting it loose some water.

4. Add the conjac noodles together with the chicken, water and soy sauce and bring to a boil, let cook for a minute or until the chicken is cooked through and the sauce reduced.

5. Turn off the heat, add the broccoli and sweet chilli sauce for seasoning (fresh ground pepper if desired) and toss everything to get covered with sauce.

6. Serve on a plate or in a large soup bowl, sprinkle with sesame seeds.

Nutrition:

Calories: 335 kcal | Carbs: 18 g | Protein: 28 g | Fat: 14 g | approximately per person

Variations:

Add roasted cashews or peanuts, honey, sweet potatoes, soy sprouts or water chestnuts. Serve with basmati rice or quinoa instead of glass noodles.

THANK YOU: My special thanks go to – alphabetically:

@alchmi of @barrel_live for the original motivational t-shirt print of my motto

@christiane.wolff for storytelling inspiration through your social media blogs

@darianinacom for publishing advice

@haribalaji.vr for inspiring me to write this book

@luke_bachmeier for nutrition coaching

@monikascheddin for inspiration through your own books and calendar

@nikkviererbl for personal training and nutrition coaching

THE AUTHOR

HANJO KOCH is a Cologne, Germany raised and Munich, Germany based hospitality industry professional with 25+ year's international experience. British educated he graduated from London South Bank University with a BA (Hons) in Hotel Management. His career lead him to work in countries like Austria, England, Germany and the United States. HANJO gained experience from privately owned properties like a heritage-site water tower turned luxury hotel, over pre-openings for major international hotel chains, to the 1000 bedroom tallest hotel in the Western Hemisphere. His fondness for sports started in early ages with basketball team sport, later extended with skiing, swimming, tennis, badminton, running and gym workouts. His professional education as a chef has helped him understand food nutrition aspects, incorporate and adapt new recipes, and enjoy cooking privately as part of an overall healthy lifestyle.

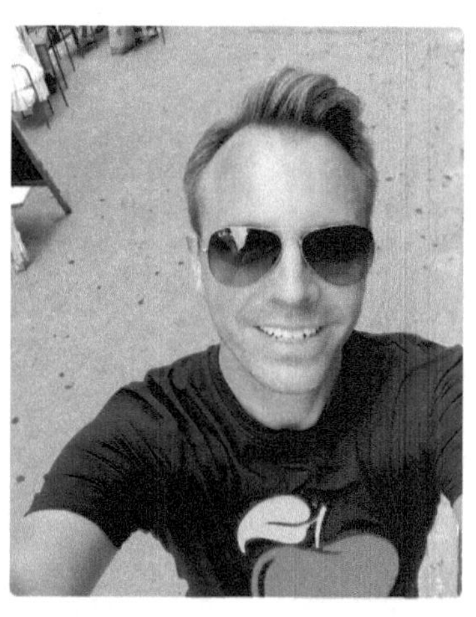

@hanjokoch | Instagram   **@hanjokochofficial | Facebook**

HANJO KOCH   Working on a new me